Dr. Michael Colgan

CREATINE
FOR
MUSCLE
AND
STRENGTH

Progressive Health Series
Colgan Institute

ISBN 1–896817–04–1

Apple Publishing Company Ltd.
220 East 59th Avenue
Vancouver, British Columbia
Canada v5x 1x9
Tel (604) 214-6688 • Fax (604) 214-3566

CONTENTS

CREATINE FOR MUSCLE AND STRENGTH

Muscle mags rave over creatine. Ads show bodybuilders bigger than bulls. Athletes declare their pecs grow so big, they have to strap 'em down so they can see to shave. You rush to buy the magic bottle. Better get two or three. You double and triple the stated dose. You train like there's no tomorrow. All you get is a net muscle loss and a niggling pain in the gut.

Am I saying that creatine is snake-oil, just like inosine, colostrum, ferrulic acid, dibencoside, glandulars and decades of other anabolic mega-scams from bee-pollen to yohimbe? No! Creatine works every time. If you're not getting good results, you're doing it wrong, dead wrong. Correct use of this boon to bodybuilding is a science. Done right, it grows muscle and strength in every man, woman, and hairy great beast we've put to the test.

YOUR ENERGY SYSTEM

To understand how creatine works, you need a thumbnail knowledge of the way you create energy. Your muscles use six overlapping fuel sources. In order of use from the moment you begin to exercise they are:

1. Adenosine Triphosphate (ATP),

2. Creatine Phosphate (CP),

3. Glycogen,

4. Glucose,

5. Fatty Acids,

6. Amino Acids.

In 1935, Sir Hans Krebs won the Nobel Prize, for his discovery of the complex chemical reactions, that convert all fuel sources to the primary energy compound—**adenosine triphosphate (ATP)**, for "burning" in the **mitochondria** ("furnaces") of your muscle cells. You begin to appreciate the power of Nature, when you realize that ATP, and only ATP, provides the energy, the life force, for all living things, from single-celled algae to human beings. It's one of the most important chemicals on earth.[1]

None of the other fuel sources operate alone to replenish ATP. Your body uses all of them together. The fuel that dominates at any moment depends on how much of it you have, and how hard and fast you work.

Because they are stored in muscles, adenosine triphosphate (ATP), creatine phosphate (CP) and glycogen are the most readily available. You can use them so quickly, they don't wait for oxygen to be delivered by the bloodstream. They are anaerobic fuels.

Glucose and fatty acids have to be delivered in the blood, so are slower to enter the energy cycle. Glucose can operate without oxygen, but fatty acids cannot. Fat-burning for fuel is always aerobic.

Amino acids for fuel come largely from the breakdown of muscle and other lean tissue proteins, a much slower process. They are also last call as an energy source, because catabolizing your body for fuel threatens its survival. Even this thumbnail biochemistry of energy, tells you exactly what form of exercise will build maximum muscle and strength.

THE ATP SYSTEM

ATP *stored* in your muscles is the only fuel instantly available for energy. Stored ATP is therefore the only fuel capable of generating 100% muscle contraction. Once stored ATP is exhausted, other fuels dominate the energy supply. Because all of them must be converted to ATP before they can be used, available energy per second declines, so maximum muscle contraction declines, also.

You can store enough ATP for about 4–5 seconds of maximum contraction, enough to do a 1-rep max squat, throw a javelin, or run 50 meters. As 100-meter sprinters know only too well, maximum muscle contraction cannot be maintained beyond 5 seconds. After that the goal is to lose as little speed as possible until you pass the finish line. This exercise requires no oxygen, and not even a molecule of carbohydrate, fat, or protein, the fuels usually cited as essential for exercise.

Because it is the only way you can ever put maximum load on your muscles, muscle contraction by stored ATP is unquestionably the most effective for building strength.[2] It creates the most extensive micro-damage, which then triggers the greatest adaptive muscle growth.

Unfortunately, it's also the most dangerous way to train, because at 100% contraction the muscle and its attachments are at greatest risk. That's why folk who are constantly pushing the max, track & field athletes, powerlifters, weightlifters, and professional athletes are always on the knife edge of muscle and connective tissue injury. Think back to the Atlanta Games. Hordes of the world's fittest and strongest were stopped cold by injury, including Leroy Burrell and Jackie Joyner Kersee. It took the genius of Bella Karoli and the indomitable will he fostered in Kerri Strug, to transcend the physiological limits of failing muscle in that once in a lifetime gold medal vault.

THE CREATINE SYSTEM

After 4–5 seconds of maximum exercise, creatine phosphate (CP) becomes the dominant energy control, permitting *near* maximum muscle contraction for another 5–6 seconds, a total of 10–11 seconds. That's enough to do a 4-rep set or sprint the 100 meters. This ATP/CP interaction is also anaerobic, and uses no glycogen, glucose, fatty acids or amino acids.

Because the ATP/CP system cannot permit maximum contraction, muscle is at less risk, so this level of exercise is much safer. Yet it still generates substantial micro-trauma, which, in turn, triggers near maximum growth. Overall, the ATP/CP 10-second window of exercise, provides the best combination of safety and efficacy for optimum strength training. Now you know why creatine is so important.

THE GLYCOGEN/GLUCOSE SYSTEM

As continuous maximum effort extends beyond 10–11 seconds, glycogen and glucose become the dominant fuel source. They permit sub-maximal performance for up to 120 seconds, enough to run 800 meters.

This is the aerobic/anaerobic edge. Oxygen becomes important, though, strictly speaking it is not essential to the chemical reactions for use of glycogen and glucose. Some aminos and fatty acids are also pulled into the fuel mix. Even though you may make maximum *effort*, muscle contraction cannot stay much above 70% of maximum for this length of time. So it's a poor way to train for muscle and strength.

THE FATTY ACID SYSTEM

For exercise longer than about 120 seconds, fatty acids begin to dominate as the fuel source. Your body also pulls a lot more amino acids into the fuel mix, providing as much as 10% of the total energy.[3] This is steady state endurance exercise, which the body can continue for many hours.

Oxygen is essential for this purely aerobic activity. It is also highly catabolic for both bodyfat and muscle. That's why you don't see muscular marathoners, and why it's not physically possible to build much strength while simultaneously training for endurance. The whole energy scenario is shown below.

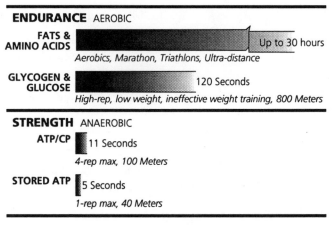

Dominant energy systems used for different types and durations of exercise done at the maximum level of muscle contraction permitted by the biochemistry of energy. © *The Colgan Institute, 1997*

HOW CREATINE WORKS

Though ATP is the life force of all living things, it's just a simple chemical, a molecule of adenosine bonded to three molecules of phosphate. By a process still completely unknown to science, a command from your brain to contract a muscle, breaks one of these phosphate bonds, causing a chemical explosion of energy. ATP is reduced to adenosine **di**phosphate (ADP), and one molecule of phosphate floats free. Creatine phosphate immediately leaps in, and regenerates the ATP by donating its own phosphate molecule, leaving a molecule of free creatine in the muscle. The ATP is then able to fire again.

Most of the free creatine and free phosphate molecules join together again to regenerate creatine phosphate. But this process requires oxygen, so you have to stop anaerobic exercise to allow it to happen. After you stop, half the spent creatine is regenerated to creatine phosphate in about 60 seconds. A maximum of 90% is regenerated within a five-minute rest period.[4] The rest is excreted from the muscles, and appears as the waste product **creatinine** in your urine.

These findings are critical for building muscle and strength, because they tell you exactly how long to rest between sets for maximum growth. In order to make the most intense muscle contraction on your next set, you have to wait until the maximum amount of creatinine has regenerated—about 4–5 minutes.

Creatine phosphate is the only way to regenerate spent ADP to ATP, and allow near maximum muscle contraction to continue past 4–5 seconds. So you can see immediately the importance of having a full load of creatine phosphate in every muscle.

SOURCES OF CREATINE

You get your creatine from two sources. First, it occurs in many foods. Best are muscle meats of animals and fish, which contain 3–6 grams of creatine per kilogram, depending on the species.[5] Your body also makes creatine in your liver, kidneys, and pancreas gland from three amino acids, the essential amino acid **methionine**, the conditionally essential amino acid **arginine**, and the nonessential amino acid **glycine**.

The average human body, however, uses over 2 grams of creatine per day, just to maintain normal energy metabolism. That's more than twice the amount in the average diet. Your body's manufacture of creatine is also limited by the intake of the amino acid, methionine, which it cannot make, and by competing calls on methionine for other tasks, such as building new proteins. For athletes the problem is compounded by the rapid use of creatine during exercise.

CREATINE UPTAKE BY MUSCLES

In 1992, Paul Greenhaff of the University of Nottingham, Queen's Medical Center in England, and Roger Harris of the Karolinska Institute in Stockholm, Sweden, and their colleagues, tested the notion that athletes may be short of creatine. They found that a 5-gram oral dose of creatine rapidly raises blood creatine levels. Increasing the dose to 5 grams, 4–6 times daily, they found a big increase in muscle creatine levels.[6]

Studies done over a century ago show that wild animals have much more creatine in their muscles than domesticated animals, a finding attributed to their greater level of exercise. [7] So Dr. Harris then made subjects exercise one leg for an hour a day. Creatine level in the exercised leg rose by another 50% more than in the unexercised leg.[6]

Recent studies confirm these findings, that oral creatine supplements increase muscle creatine, and that strenuous exercise increases muscle uptake of creatine by about another 50%.[7,8,9]. So it's likely that most athletes have suboptimal levels of creatine in their muscles.

CREATINE FOR STRENGTH

The chemistry of creatine tells us just what we might expect from supplementation. For short, intense exercise beyond about 5 seconds, extra muscle creatine should regenerate more ATP, therefore permitting more intense muscle contraction. So as soon as your muscles are loaded with creatine, you should be stronger right away.

Recent research dramatically supports this hypothesis. At Nottingham University in England, Paul Greenhaff and colleagues gave cyclists 4 doses of 5 grams of creatine per day for 5 days and compared them with a placebo. Creatine increased peak power output by a huge 6% during a 30-second maximum effort.[7]

At the Karolinska Institute in Sweden, Paul Balsom and colleagues tested male subjects on the cycle ergometer using 5 sets of 6 seconds at a fixed work intensity, with 30-second rest periods. After another 40 seconds, they did a 10-second maximum effort. Then he gave them 20 grams of creatine per day for six days and tested them again. Creatine supplementation increased work output during the maximum effort by 5%.[9]

In the most recent study, Conrad Earnest and colleagues at Texas Southwestern Medical Center and The Cooper Clinic in Dallas, gave experienced weight trainers 20 grams of creatine per day for 28 days. They measured performance on the 1-rep maximum bench press. The average increase was 18 lbs, a 6.5% improvement in strength.[11]

Because of cost and logistics, all these controlled studies are short- term. At the Colgan Institute we have made careful long-term measurements of strength improvements in case studies of elite track and field athletes, and bodybuilders, using creatine cycles for periods of more than two years. With four 8-week cycles per year, separated by rests of 4 weeks, we've found strength increases in the 1-rep maximum squat of almost 20% in a year. Because these athletes are already at the top end of the strength curve, — that's enormous! A 500 lb. squat increases to 600 lbs! If you do creatine the right way, you can't miss.

MUSCLE GROWTH

The second prediction from the biochemistry of creatine, is that supplementation will allow you to carry on near maximal exercise for longer, so you should be able to train harder, and therefore generate faster muscle growth.

In the strength study above, Dr. Earnest found that average repetitions at 70% of 1-rep maximum increased from 11 to 15.[11] Paul Balsom and team at the Karolinska Institute also found a significant increase in work output. They tested subjects over 10 sets of 6-second bouts of cycling at two levels of high intensity. Compared with a placebo group, creatine increased the amount of work done at both levels.[12]

This study is a good model of intermittent heavyweight, low-rep exercise that characterizes the best weight training. By increasing muscle overload the most, it stimulates the greatest adaptive growth. And plenty of growth there was. Over a one-month period Dr. Balsom found increases in lean mass of 0.7 to 5.5 lbs., with an average of 2.4 lbs.[12] Conrad Earnest found even greater growth in his studies. After 28 days of 20 grams of creatine per day, his subjects showed an average increase in lean mass of 3.5 lbs.[11]

In a more recent study in 1995, Balsom reports similar increases in mass in *six days* of 20 grams creatine per day.[8] You may see these figures cited in ads, but give them no respect. At the Colgan Institute we have seen similar jumps in bodyweight, only to find later they were mostly water. But 2.4 – 3.5 lbs. over one month is a good bet for real lean tissue growth, and is beyond anything a drug-free athlete can achieve without creatine. It makes believable the claim of beautiful fitness model and TV host, Marla Duncan, that she gained 10 lbs. of lean mass over a year of creatine supplementation.[13]

CREATINE AIDS RECOVERY

During exercise beyond about 11 seconds, glycogen, glucose, and then fatty acids become the dominant fuels. A by-product of their conversion to ATP is **lactic acid**. Lactic acid lowers the pH of muscles into the acid range, and inactivates crucial enzymes that enable the muscles to use glycogen, glucose, and fat for fuel. It's the main component of the burn that stops you exercising at the end of every set, and prevents you beginning another set until it dissipates, mainly by conversion back to ATP.

Extra creatine phosphate in the muscle reduces use of other fuels. It also acts as an acid buffer. It should therefore inhibit lactic acid build-up, enabling you to exercise longer and recover faster. This effect should occur most in short-duration high-intensity exercise, such as weightlifting, that put greatest demands on the creatine phosphate system.

The evidence supports all these hypotheses. In their 1993 study discussed above, Paul Balsom and colleagues found reduced lactic acid levels after creatine supplementation.[12] In their 1995 study of repeated bouts of 6-second exercise at fixed intensity, creatine caused a 41% reduction in lactic acid. After a 10-second maximum effort, lactic acid was still 18% lower than before supplementation.

In longer-duration exercise, however, creatine shows little effect on lactic acid. Michael Stroud and colleagues at Nottingham University gave subjects 20 grams of creatine per day for five days and then made them run for 7 sets of 6-minutes on the treadmill, increasing from 50% to 90% of VO2 max (the subject's maximal oxygen uptake). Lactic acid levels were similar before and after creatine supplementation.[14]

Some researchers take these results to mean that creatine has no effect on endurance performance. They are mistaken. Because stored creatine dramatically reduces glycogen use during the first minute of exercise, it must therefore leave more glycogen to fuel subsequent exercise.

The problem lies in the sensitivity of measurement of studies that have to rely on group averages. As exercise duration increases, stored muscle creatine represents a progressively smaller percentage of total fuel used. So it's effect on performance becomes increasingly difficult to detect, using statistics which have to rely on significant percentage differences between groups.

A further indication that creatine aids short-term recovery is your blood level of **ammonia**, a toxic by-product of energy metabolism that increases rapidly when ATP becomes depleted. As I documented in **Optimum Sports Nutrition**, ammonia devastates performance.[3] The 1993 Greenhaff study above, found a significant reduction in ammonia with creatine supplementation. So did a 1994 study by Steven Birch and team at Nottingham University, using 30-second sets of cycling at maximum effort.[10] Overall, the evidence to date, strongly supports the use of creatine to aid recovery in short, intense exercise, just the sort of training that yields the best muscle growth.

HOW MUCH CREATINE?

The daily intake of creatine you need for maximum effect on muscle and strength depends on how much muscle you have to fill. It also depends on how much exercise you do. If you are keen enough to study this article, I'm assuming that you are training at high intensity, that is 5-days per week or more. If you're not training that hard, then increasing your training will have more effect than creatine or any other ergogenic supplement, so don't waste your money. Studies show that resistance exercise an hour a day raises muscle creatine the most.[6] To get the benefits from creatine you have to train!

Some guides to creatine use, use bodyweight to calculate creatine need.[13] It's a poor measure because folk vary widely in bodyfat. Bodyfat doesn't need creatine. Over 95% of body creatine is in your muscles. At the Colgan Institute we use muscle weight as the major criterion.

As I've shown before in MD, muscle weight in athletes is about 50% of lean weight in men and 35% of lean weight in women. So, in order to find out your personal creatine requirement, you have to know your **lean weight**, that is, your bodyweight minus your fat weight.

Some ignorant guys I meet, who are so small inside they need to constantly exhibit their machismo say, "To hell with the science crap. So-and-so (hero) is taking 30 grams a day, so I am too."

Don't! Excess creatine whacks your liver and kidneys, which have to get rid of it. You will also get acute diarrhea, which is one of the best known ways to *lose* muscle.

In a recent study at the Karolinska Institute, Roger Harris and team, gave subjects 30 grams of creatine per day and measured the amount excreted. He didn't calculate lean mass, but average weight of subjects was 175 lbs (82 kg). Under a light exercise regimen, their bodies excreted 40% of the creatine on Day 1, rising to 68% by Day 3.[6] So most of the creatine was being converted to waste. No one knows how much damage this might do to your kidneys long-term, but it's likely to be substantial. If you want fully functioning kidneys in later life, don't overload creatine. If you have kidney problems now, don't use creatine at all.

CREATINE LOADING AND MAINTENANCE

Studies in the early '90s found that low doses of creatine didn't raise muscle creatine much.[6] We have found the same results for blood creatine levels in single case studies. So there's some justification for loading creatine at the beginning of a cycle. Whether this strategy is essential to trigger super-loading of the muscles, is still being investigated. Until the evidence is out, loading is in.

After reviewing all studies to date, we adopted a 6-day creatine loading regimen, using 0.5 grams of creatine per kilogram *muscle* weight. To save you the sums, the daily amount of creatine for loading, based on your **lean** weight, and high intensity training, is given in the table on the next page.

CREATINE LOADING AND MAINTENANCE

Lean Bodyweight		Males		Females	
WEIGHT LBS	WEIGHT KG	LOADING GMS	MAINTENANCE GMS	LOADING GMS	MAINTENANCE GMS
80	36	9	3	6	2
100	45	11	3.5	8	2.5
120	55	14	4.5	10	3
140	64	16	5	11.5	3.5
160	73	18	6	13	4
180	82	20	6.5	14.5	4.5
200	91	22.5	7	16	5
220	100	25	8	17.5	6

Source: © The Colgan Institute, San Diego, 1996.

Once you are loaded, it doesn't take a lot of creatine to keep you there. There's some evidence from Paul Balsom that subjects at unspecified levels of exercise, need only 10% of the loading dose.[9] In case studies of athletes exercising at high intensity, we have found this amount insufficient. Until better controlled evidence comes out, we have adopted 25% of the loading dose as the maintenance criterion. Maintenance doses are also given in the table. That's all the creatine you'll ever need.

USE CREATINE RIGHT

Creatine monohydrate is the only supplement form of creatine that is reasonable stable. it is a white, gritty, odorless, tasteless powder. Open a capsule and try it. If you sense any taste or smell, then it is degraded or contaminated, or perhaps not creatine at all, and definitely will not work.

There's a lot of inferior creatine about. As with all supplements, buy only from a firm with a reputation to lose. Firms with no reputation, or who have lost their reputation, have nothing to gain by making quality, because no one will believe them anyway. So they have nothing more to lose by continuing to make garbage.

Once you have a good creatine source, and have worked out your personal daily dose from the Table above, you still have a few things to do to ensure optimum results. You want maximum absorption and maximum transport of creatine into the muscles. Here's how to get it.

DIVIDED DOSES

The first strategy to load creatine is, divided doses, taken at spaced intervals throughout the day. Divide your daily intake into four. Take one dose 30–60 minutes before workout. Creatine is then digested and in the bloodstream by the time you begin exercise. As the muscles use creatine rapidly, you get a small absorption edge by having plenty available.

Take anther dose immediately after workout. After exercise your muscles are hungry for creatine. so if you get into the bloodstream within 30 minutes after workout, you get a further edge in muscle uptake. Take the other two doses spaced out to fill the day.

SUGAR IS ESSENTIAL

The second strategy is sugar. You enhance muscle uptake of creatine by taking each dose with an 8 oz drink containing 30-40 grams of mixed sugars. The sugars stimulate the insulin that is essential to push creatine through muscle cell membranes.

We use a 50:50 mix of grape juice and grapefruit juice. Grapefruit juice contains an enzyme that reduces stomach acidity. There is also some evidence that it enhances absorption of many compounds by an independent mechanism. Dextrose and maltodextrin drinks also work but don't have these added advantages.

BOOST INSULIN EFFICIENCY

The next strategy is to maximize insulin efficiency. In almost all the research and in some case studies at the Colgan Institute, some individuals showed increased blood creatine levels, but no increase in muscle or strength. Various researchers usages this failure may be caused by inefficient insulin metabolism,[13] or insulin resistance,[11] whereby insulin fails in its normal task of moving chemicals through the cell membrane.

When we examined the nutrition and blood profiles of our non-responders, we found two prominent problems. First, most of their diets contained insufficient chromium for normal insulin metabolism. Many of them also showed somewhat elevated blood sugar, blood insulin, and blood triglycerides, the classic symptom trilogy of insulin resistance. When we added 400-800 mcg of chromium picolinate, and 300–600 mg of omega-3 fatty acids to the creatine mix, most of our failures became successes. Both chromium picolinate and omega-3 fatty acids are well established potentiators of insulin metabolism.)[14,15]

In more recent cases, we have also used 25 mg of dehydroepiandrosterone (DHEA). Levels of this hormone begin to decline after age 20, and recent research shows that supplementation with 25 mg per day, restores youthful levels and enhances insulin efficiency.[16]

CYCLE CREATINE

Finally, you should cycle creatine. No one knows whether continuous creatine supplementation interferes with the body's own ability to make creatine, or whether the human body adapts to the supplements over long-term use, so that muscle creatine declines at its former level. Until that research is done, we cycle creatine over 8 weeks with a 4-week rest.

As with all supplements that have big effects on body function, where evidence of long-term safety is lacking, we treat the chemical with respect. You should too. If you follow this article to help you use creatine, you should first read the scientific references. Even then, you use it at your own choice and risk.

Over five years of using creatine with healthy folk, beyond occasional diarrhea and stomach upset, we have found no side-effects. Our usual experience is a much improved athlete, smiling ear-to-ear.

Michael Colgan
San Diego, California, 1997

REFERENCES

1. Stryer L. **Biochemistry, 2nd Ed**. New York: W.H. Freeman, 1981.

2. Colgan M. **The Power Program**. San Diego: CI Publications, 1991.

3. Colgan M. **Optimum Sports Nutrition**, New York: Advanced Research Press, 1993.

4. Soderlund K, Hultman E. ATP and phosphcreatine changes in single human muscle fibers after intense electrical stimulation. **Amer J Physiol**, 1991: 261:E737-E741.

5. McCance RA, Widdowson EM. **Composition Of Foods, 5th Ed**. Cambridge: Royal Society of Chemistry, 1991

6. Harris R, et al. Elevation of creatine in resting and exercise muscles of normal subjects by creatine supplementation. **Clin Sci**, 1992:83:367-374.

7. Greenhaff P. Creatine and its application as an ergogenic aid. **Int J Sports Nutr**, 1995:5:S100-S110.

8. Balsom PD, et al. Skeletal muscle metabolism during short duration, high intensity exercise: influence of creatine supplementation. **Acta Physiol Scand**, 1995:154:303-310

9. Balsom P, et al. Creatine in humans with special reference to creatine supplementation. **Sports Med**, 1994:18:268-280.

10. Birch R, et al. The influence of dietary creatine supplementation on performance during repeated bouts of maximal isokinetic cycling in man. **Eur J Appl Physiol**, 1994:69:268-276.

11. Earnest C, et al. The effect of creatine monohydrate ingestion on anaerobic power indices, muscular strength and body composition. **Acta Physiol Scand**, 1995: 153:207-209.

12. Balsom P, et al. Creatine supplementation and dynamic high-intensity intermittent exercise. **Scand J Med Sci Sports**, 1993;3:143-149.

13. Sahelian R, Tuttle D. **Creatine: Nature's Muscle Builder**. New York: Avery Publishing, 1997.

14. Storlien, LH. **Science,** 1987;237:885

15. Evans, GW. The effect of chromium picolinate on insulin controlled parameters in humans. **Int J Biosocial Med Res**, 1989;11:163-180.

16. Colgan M. **Hormonal Health**, Vancouver: Apple Publishing, 1996.

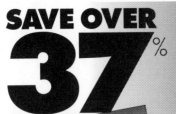
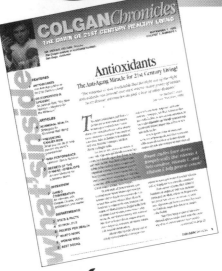

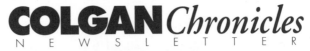